WAY GROSS SCIENCE™

THE GROSS SCIENCE OF BAD BREATH AND CAVITIES

JESSICA SHAW

rosen publishing's rosen central®
New York

Published in 2019 by The Rosen Publishing Group, Inc.
29 East 21st Street, New York, NY 10010

First Edition

Library of Congress Cataloging-in-Publication Data

Names: Shaw, Jessica, 1972– author.
Title: The gross science of bad breath and cavities / Jessica Shaw.
Description: New York : Rosen Central, 2019. | Series: Way gross science | Audience: Grades 5–8. | Includes bibliographical references and index.
Identifiers: LCCN 2017045969| ISBN 9781508181620 (library bound) | ISBN 9781508181637 (pbk.)
Subjects: LCSH: Bad breath—Causes—Juvenile literature. | Mouth—Diseases—Juvenile literature. | Mouth—Care and hygiene—Juvenile literature. | Teeth—Diseases—Juvenile literature. | Teeth—Care and hygiene—Juvenile literature.
Classification: LCC RC815 .S4585 2019 | DDC 616.3/1—dc23
LC record available at https://lccn.loc.gov/2017045969

Manufactured in the United States of America

CONTENTS

INTRODUCTION

More than 2,100 years ago in Egypt, a man was suffering extreme pain due to his many cavities and abscesses. He was young, in his late twenties or early thirties, and was wealthy enough to afford the services of a dentist. His abscesses—large, infected, pus-filled sacs between his teeth and gums—probably stank almost as bad as they felt. Though this man's cavities and abscesses were very extreme, dental problems were a common occurrence in the area because the ancient Egyptians ate a coarsely ground grain that was bad for their teeth. Unfortunately, even though dentistry had been practiced in Egypt since at least as far back as when the Great Pyramids were built around 2500 BCE, not much was known about preventing or treating cavities and abscesses. All the money in the world could not buy the necessary treatment, and despite the dentist's best efforts, the man died and was then mummified.

In 1859, a young businessman and politician named James Ferrier brought this man's mummified remains from Egypt to Montreal, Canada, to be studied. Advances in technology have given scientists the ability to closely examine the mummy's teeth and body. Using images obtained from a high-resolution CT scanner, they determined the man was suffering greatly before his death. His cavities and abscesses had caused a severe sinus infection, which may have been what ultimately caused his death. The images showed that the dentist did his best, but lacked in both knowledge and equipment. The man's largest and worst cavity was in one of his molars and had been packed with a piece of linen between it and the next tooth. Researchers believe the linen was most likely soaked in something like cedar oil or fig juice, in an attempt to ease the man's pain.

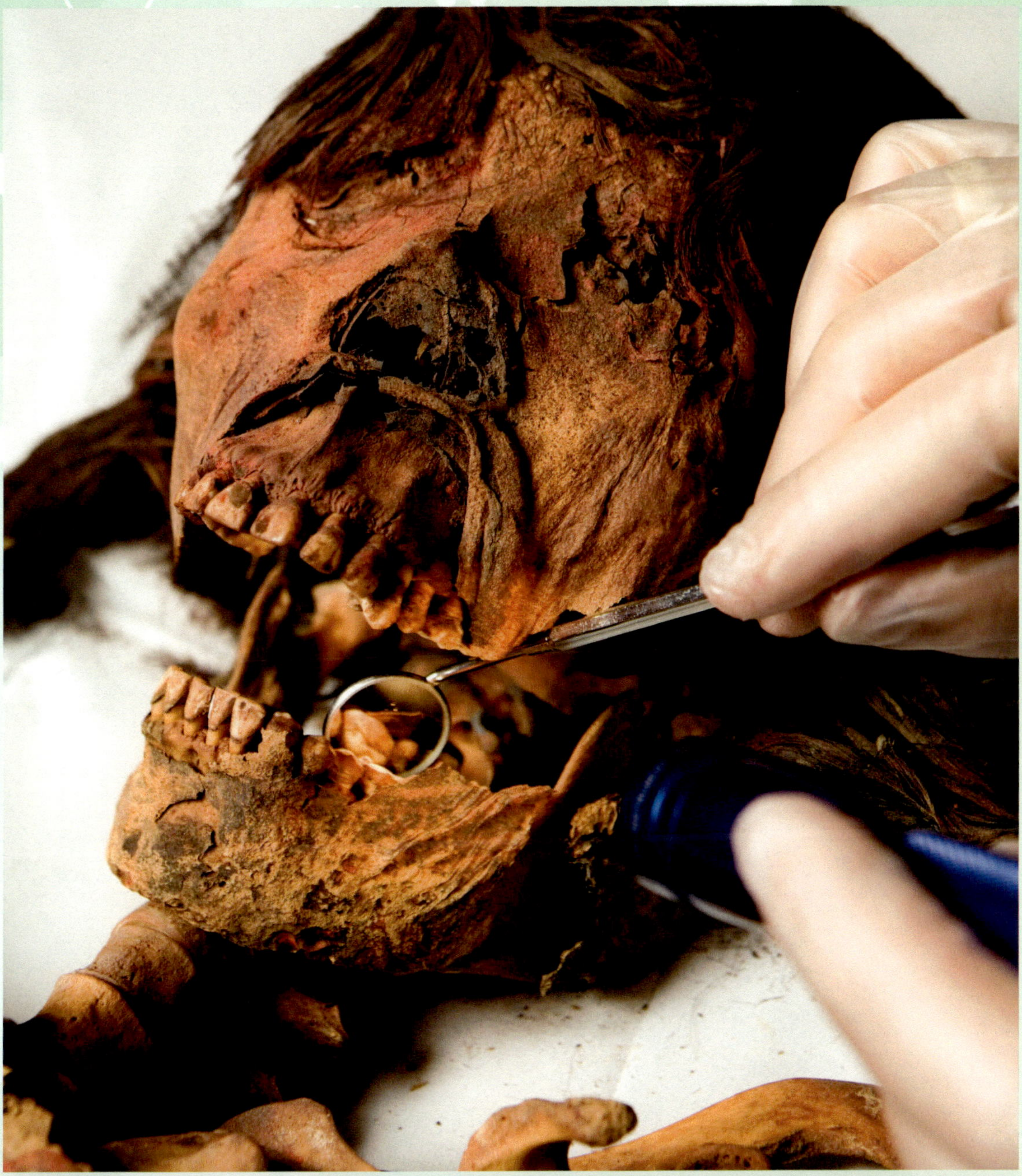

Through the study of ancient, mummified remains, scientists have discovered that people have suffered and sought relief from tooth decay for thousands of years.

There is proof of terrible tooth decay in people who lived long before the unfortunate mummified man. Fifteen thousand years ago, a community of hunter-gatherers lived in a large cave in Morocco. Their diet consisted primarily of meat from animals they caught, but they also ate a sweet variety of acorns. When scientists studied the remains of fifty-two people buried in the cave, they found that forty-nine of them had several cavities. Some of them had bad abscesses and tooth decay so advanced that the top part of their teeth—the crown—had come off, which meant they were chewing on the exposed roots of their teeth. It was not the meat in their diet, but the acorns, that caused their dental problems. They boiled the acorns, which made them soft and gooey...perfect for sticking to teeth and allowing bacteria to eat away at the enamel. With only primitive toothpicks to clean their teeth, most of these people developed multiple cavities and experienced severe pain in their mouths for weeks, months, even years before they died.

Today, most people have the items necessary to keep their teeth clean and prevent cavities. When issues such as chronic bad breath, tooth decay, or any other oral hygiene problems arise, there are qualified, well-trained dentists and dental hygienists who can help, but toothpaste, mouthwash, dental floss, and proper dental treatment did not come about until the late 1800s. The mummified man who endured unspeakable pain in his final days and weeks more than 2,100 years ago has a lot to teach people about the value of practicing good oral hygiene—and being grateful for modern-day dentistry!

CHAPTER ONE

THE HISTORY OF TREATING FOUL MOUTHS

Bad breath and cavities have plagued people since the beginning of recorded history. All kinds of cures and treatments have been invented over thousands of years to try to treat cavities or cover up foul-smelling breath. Some of these treatments actually helped, some didn't make much of a difference at all, and some were just plain disgusting!

EARLY METHODS OF TREATING BAD BREATH AND CAVITIES

One of the earliest breath mints was invented by the ancient Egyptians about three thousand years ago. They boiled herbs and spices, including frankincense, myrrh, and cinnamon, and mixed them with honey to make a type of candy that could be chewed on or sucked. They didn't realize that having that concoction of spices and sweet, sticky honey in their mouths was most likely causing further tooth decay, even if it temporarily masked the bad odor.

Those who were especially desperate to get rid of their bad breath might have taken the advice given by a Roman author known as Pliny the Elder in his book, *Natural History*, published around 77 CE. Pliny

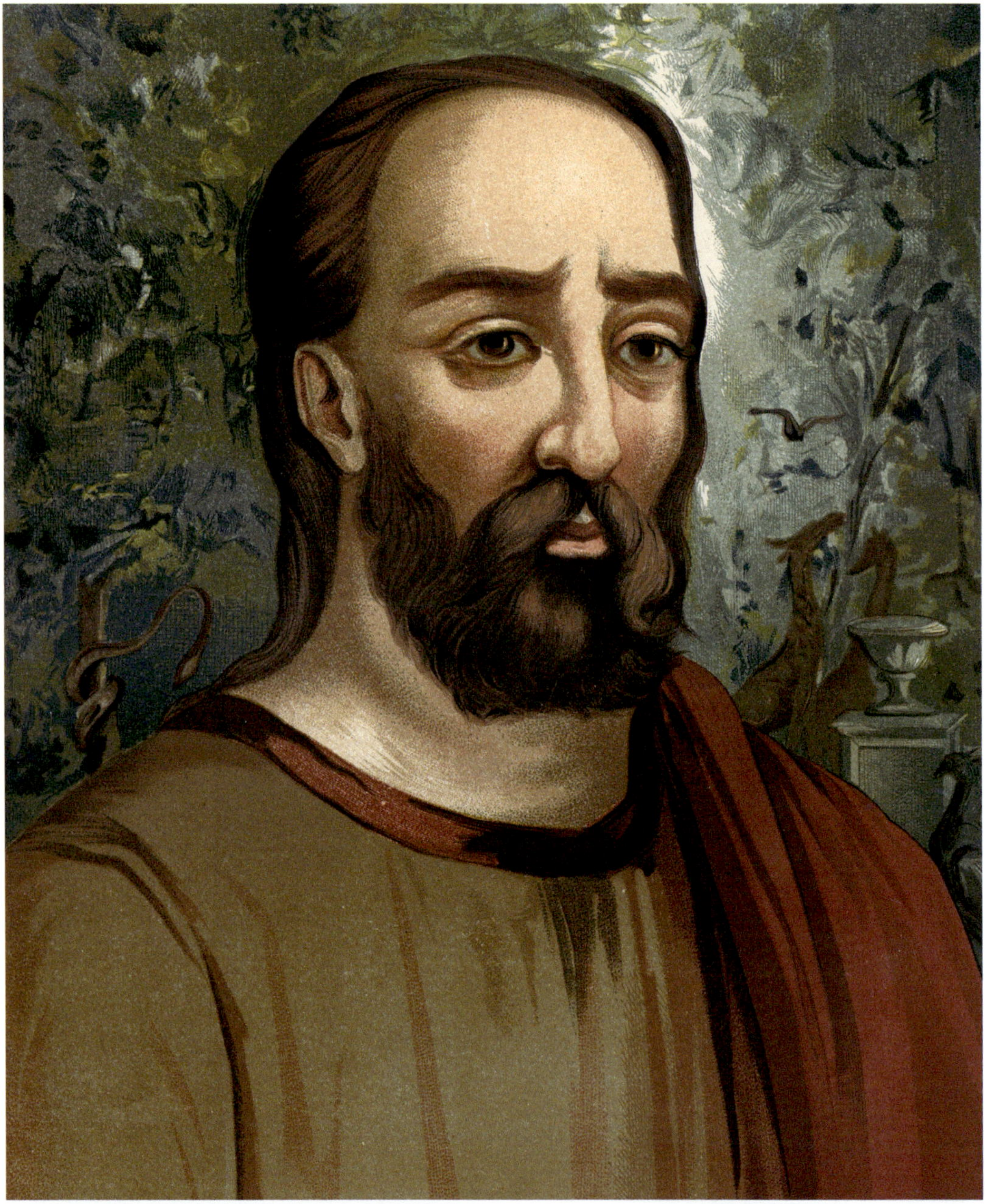

During the first century, Roman author Pliny the Elder dished out some truly disgusting advice for those trying to cure their bad breath.

the Elder's suggestions for sweetening the breath included picking one's teeth with porcupine quills and rubbing the teeth with the ashes of burnt mouse dung and honey!

Another early popular choice for taking care of bad breath that was not nearly as disgusting as the mouse dung was using chewing gum made from tree resin. Though they didn't know it at the time, testing has proven the resin has antibacterial properties. This antibacterial tree-resin gum is still used in Greece and Turkey today.

Based on studies done at archaeological sites, scientists think prehistoric humans tried out several different methods of treating dental problems, including drilling out rotted cavities, sealing tooth fractures with beeswax, and removing rotted teeth. They believe the thirteen-thousand-year-old skeletal remains of a person in Italy may be the oldest known example of an attempt at tooth fillings. There were holes in the person's two front teeth that went all the way from the surface to the inner pulp of the teeth. There were scratch marks inside the holes, from a tool of some sort that was used to remove the cavities. Inside the holes were traces of a tarlike substance called bitumen that was used to fill the cavities.

Beginning in the 1930s, companies selling mouthwash and other products to improve breath began running newspaper and magazine ads that pointed out the embarrassment of having bad breath in social situations. This type of advertising played on people's fears of being excluded or gossiped about. Many people purchased the advertised products rather than talking to a dentist about their problem.

THE EVOLUTION OF THE TOOTHBRUSH

Early attempts at cleaning the teeth can be traced back thousands of years. Around 3500 BCE, Egyptians and Babylonians used sticks to clean their teeth. They chewed on one end until it became soft and frayed, like a brush, and they kept the other end pointed, to pick out food that was

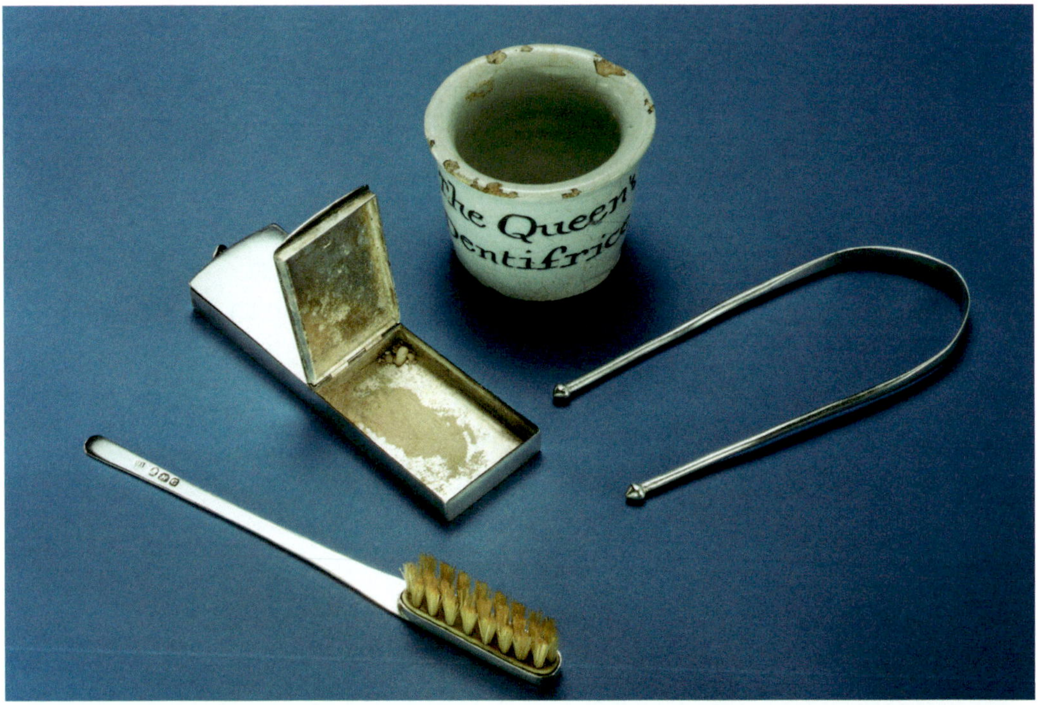

Dental tools of the eighteenth century included crude toothbrushes, dental powder, and metal tongue scrapers.

stuck between their teeth. In China, similar chewing sticks were used in 1600 BCE.

Finally, in fifteenth-century China, the first tooth cleaning tool with a handle and bristles was invented. Bamboo or animal bone was used for the handle, and stiff hog hair was used for the bristles. This invention soon caught on in Europe as well, and by the eighteenth century, the first mass-produced toothbrushes, made from cattle bone and pig fibers, were being sold in England.

The toothbrush continued to evolve, and in the 1930s, the pig fibers were replaced with the nylon bristles used on our modern-day toothbrushes. Today, people have many features to choose from when buying a toothbrush. There are handles with special grips, many sizes

TWO COUSINS AND ONE "CRAZY" IDEA

Dr. Alfred Fones, a young dentist from Connecticut, was one of the early crusaders for preventive dentistry and the training of dental hygienists. In 1906, he took time out from his full schedule of dental extractions to begin training his cousin Irene Newman to clean patients' teeth. She began working on patients in his office in 1907. Many thought the idea that people would go to a dentist to have their teeth cleaned was crazy. At the time, dentist visits were typically just for having teeth pulled. Still, Dr. Fones believed in the idea of keeping teeth clean to reduce bacteria in the mouth and prevent cavities.

Newman became skilled at cleaning teeth and is known as the first practicing dental hygienist. By 1917, the cousins had begun training the first dental hygienist students, with people from as far away as Japan traveling to Connecticut to learn from them. The pair also began a school program to teach children how to properly clean their teeth. Irene Newman was the first person to be issued a license for practicing dental hygiene, and the efforts of Fones and Newman inspired similar programs across the United States. People's views about the importance of good oral hygiene and the value of skilled professionals trained to properly clean teeth were forever changed thanks to two cousins who pursued one "crazy idea."

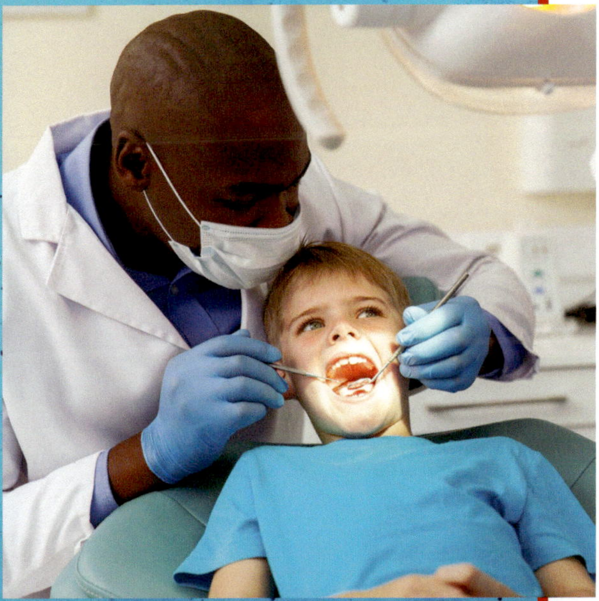

Regular dental checkups and cleanings have proven highly effective in preventing cavities, gum disease, and related health problems.

and shapes of toothbrush heads, varying softness in the bristles, and even electric toothbrushes...and the best part is that no one has to put hog bristles in his or her mouth!

THE INTRODUCTION OF DENTAL HYGIENISTS

As teeth cleaning tools and methods continued to advance, so did the field of dentistry. People began to realize the importance of preventing dental problems, rather than just treating them. The first "dental nurses" began assisting dentists with prophylactic treatment—treatment to prevent disease of the teeth and gums—in the 1880s. By the early 1900s, many dentists referred to their "dental nurses" as "dental hygienists," but there was no school or formal training for these positions.

Dr. C. M. Wright of Cincinnati, Ohio, was one of the first dentists to try to bring about a big change in the field of dentistry. He knew that dental hygienists could make the difference between a mouth full of stinky, rotted teeth and a mouth full of clean, healthy teeth. In 1902, he published a paper asking dental colleges to offer special lectures and training for dental hygienists. His hope was that after the special training, dental hygienists would earn a dental college certificate, which would qualify them for employment with dentists. Despite Wright's efforts, it was not until 1917 that Connecticut became the first state to pass a dental hygiene licensure law. Over the next several decades, more and more states began to offer dental hygienist training programs and require hygienists to obtain a license before working in the field of dentistry. By 1952, all states in the United States offered licensure programs for dental hygienists.

CHAPTER TWO

BAD BREATH STINKS

No one wants to have bad breath, but it's estimated that one in four people in the world suffer from it on a regular basis. Bad breath can keep people from socializing, make work or school interactions difficult, and cause shame and embarrassment. It's a serious problem for a lot of people, and yet many of them try to deal with it on their own rather than seeking professional help from a dentist.

WHAT IS HALITOSIS?

Halitosis is the scientific term for persistent bad breath. Bacteria are tiny, living organisms that are too small to see without a microscope. There are hundreds of different species and millions of bacteria, good and bad, inside everyone's mouth, especially on the surface of the tongue and in the tissue below the gumline. Living organisms need to eat, and bacteria enjoy feasting on the particles of food and tissue inside the mouth. As they munch away on those tidbits, different types of bacteria cause different breath odors by creating smelly chemical compounds. One of those compounds, hydrogen sulfide, is responsible for rotten egg odor. Another, putrescine, gives off the aroma of rotten meat. Certain foods, such as those classified as carbohydrates, make a perfect meal for many of the odor-causing, "bad" bacteria. The "good" bacteria, on the

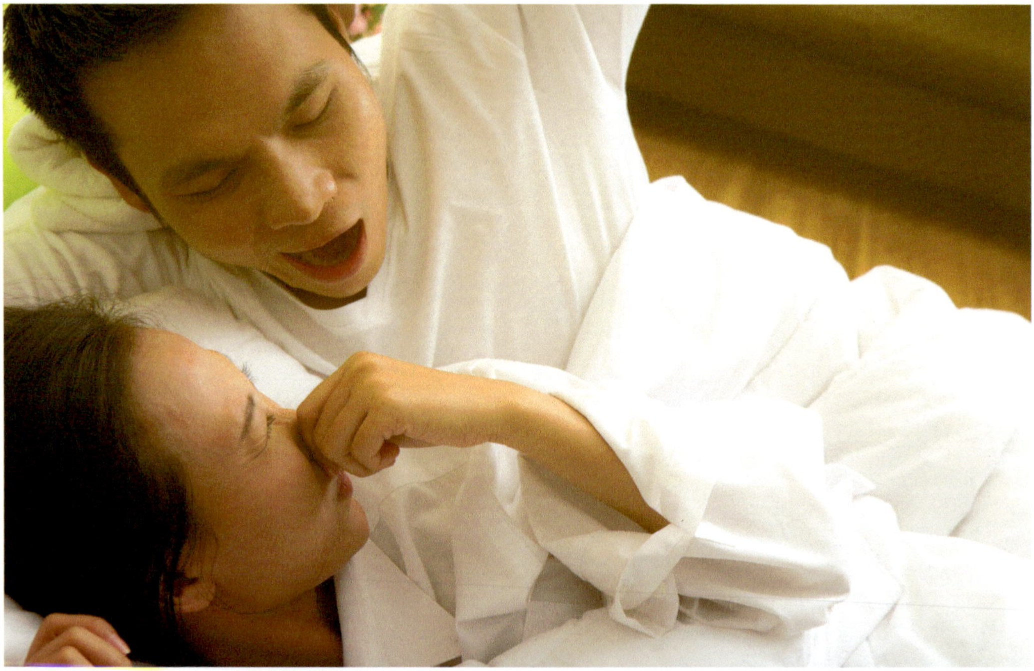

An overabundance of "bad" bacteria in the mouth, eating foods such as garlic and onions, and a lack of proper oral hygiene can all contribute to bad breath.

other hand, are important for a healthy mouth. They keep the number of bad bacteria in balance and perform a variety of other functions to help improve digestion and overall health. When the bad bacteria in the mouth outnumber and overpower the good bacteria, one of the results is bad breath that just won't go away.

BAD BREATH CULPRITS

Though oral bacteria are largely to blame for bad breath, they need help making the breath as nasty as possible. The thing that helps them the most is poor oral hygiene. In other words, people who don't properly brush their teeth, floss, or visit a dentist regularly are rolling out the red

FOODS THAT FIGHT BAD BREATH

Most people know there are certain foods that make breath odor worse, and many even avoid eating those foods when they are out in public to prevent foul-smelling breath. There are some types of food and drink, however, which actually help to fight bad breath. One of the simplest ways to prevent stinky breath is to drink plenty of water after eating to wash away bits of food clinging to the teeth. Having a piece of cheese or some unsweetened yogurt after eating a meal has been shown to reduce some of the acids in food and the levels of hydrogen sulfide, a compound that contributes to bad breath. Drinking black tea also prevents the growth of bacteria that causes bad breath. Eating crunchy snacks such as carrots or apples is another way to eliminate sticky food particles on the teeth that could feed the bacteria and lead to bad odor. Finally, sugar-free candy or gum increases saliva in the mouth, which also helps fight odor. With mouths full of stink-causing bacteria and many foods that turn harmless breath into horrible breath, it's good to know there are recipes for success in the struggle to keep breath sweet!

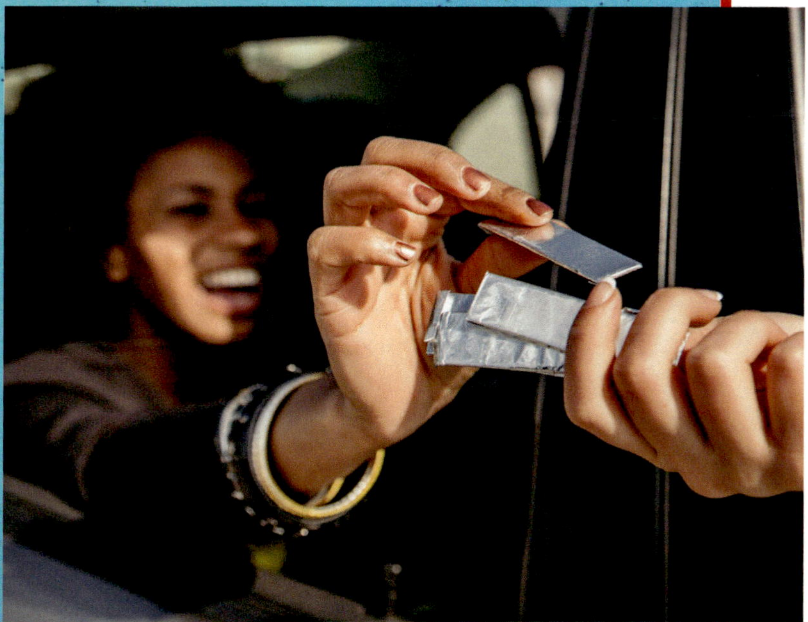

Many people use mouthwash, mints, and sugar-free chewing gum in an attempt to eliminate bad breath.

carpet for all the bad bacteria in their mouths. Excessive bad bacteria that forms a thick layer on the teeth is known as plaque. Plaque is clear or white in color and difficult to brush or floss away if it gets out of hand. The thicker the plaque, the more bacteria, and the harder it is to get rid of bad breath. If not removed, the bacteria in plaque causes cavities, and as a cavity worsens, it gives off foul-smelling gases such as hydrogen sulfide. Aside from poor oral hygiene, there are many other culprits that also play a role in promoting halitosis. Some of these bad breath boosters are easier to stop than others. Certain foods, such as garlic and onions, are known for causing bad breath. When they are digested, they absorb into the bloodstream, travel to the lungs, and then become bad breath. Having a dry mouth means there is not enough saliva in the mouth. Saliva helps wash away bacteria, so when the mouth is dry, bad breath is

THE TRUTH ABOUT HALITOSIS

Those who suffer from halitosis often use a lot of breath mints and mouthwash in an attempt to cure their bad breath. The truth is, breath mints and mouthwash only mask bad breath and usually only for a few minutes. Mouthwash does help to kill bacteria in the mouth, but mouthwashes that are made with alcohol dry out the mouth, which makes bad breath even worse. Another misconception is that brushing numerous times throughout the day will eliminate bad breath. Regular brushing is important, but brushing too frequently can not only damage the gums and teeth, it also dries out the mouth, which makes halitosis worse. Fortunately, there are methods that have proven very effective for keeping chronic bad breath under control. A visit to the dentist is the best place to start when bad breath just won't go away.

more likely. Using tobacco products can cause seriously nasty breath, not to mention many other health problems. Though rare, halitosis can also be caused by certain medical conditions, such as sinus infections, some cancers, or liver failure.

PREVENTING AND TREATING BAD BREATH

Most people realize that brushing and flossing are important daily activities that help keep breath odor free. However, a surprising number

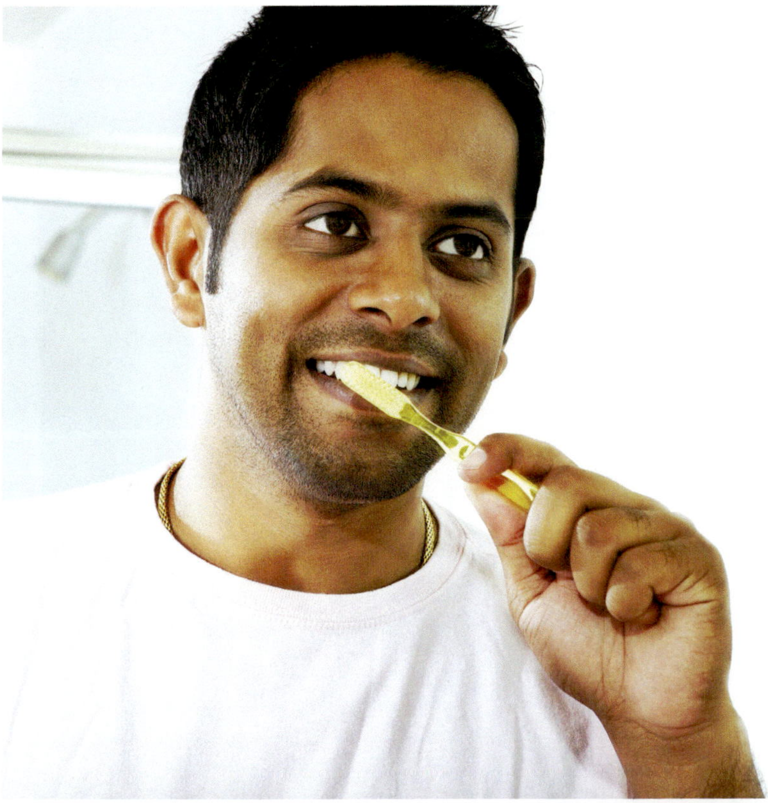

Using proper technique when brushing and flossing is essential to maintaining a clean, healthy mouth. Brush and floss daily.

of people may be brushing and flossing incorrectly. Proper brushing begins with a fluoride toothpaste and a quality soft-bristled toothbrush. Technique is very important for removing sticky plaque and food particles. Teeth should be brushed with short back-and-forth motions at least twice a day, on all surfaces: outside, inside, and chewing surfaces.

Even though it may look clean, scientists have found that a single toothbrush can be home to more than ten million bacteria, along with viruses. Over time, the bacteria multiply in the moist bristles of the brush, and the bristles become worn and ineffective. For these reasons, toothbrushes should be replaced at least every three months. In addition to brushing, floss should be used between all teeth every day. Bacteria can thrive in the spaces between teeth, especially if plaque and bits of food are not removed with floss. Visiting a dentist twice a year for a professional cleaning is ideal. Limiting foods that may stick to the teeth, using mouthwash every day, and brushing or scraping the surface of the tongue are other ways to cut down on odor-causing bacteria and maintain a healthy mouth.

CHAPTER THREE

CAVITIES ARE ROTTEN

The same bacteria that cause bad breath can lead to a potentially much more serious problem. Tooth decay is damage that occurs when the bacteria make acids that eat away at the tooth enamel. This can lead to cavities, tooth loss, and even serious infections.

CAVITIES AND THEIR CAUSES

So what exactly is a cavity? Simply put, a cavity is a hole in a tooth caused by decay. When the amount of harmful bacteria in the mouth overpowers the good bacteria, the amount of plaque on teeth increases. After eating, the bacteria in plaque interact with the food particles and create acid that attacks the teeth. Over time, these attacks wear down the surface of the tooth. Eventually, if the teeth are not properly cleaned on a regular basis, the enamel rots away and a hole—a cavity—forms. Cavities can occur on any surface of a tooth: the eating surface, the inner or outer side of a tooth, or the often-neglected tight space in between teeth. Plaque that isn't brushed or flossed away and remains on the teeth for an extended period of time becomes hard and turns yellow or brown. This hardened plaque is called tartar. Once plaque turns into tartar, it not only continues to eat away at tooth enamel, it is also too hard to be removed by brushing

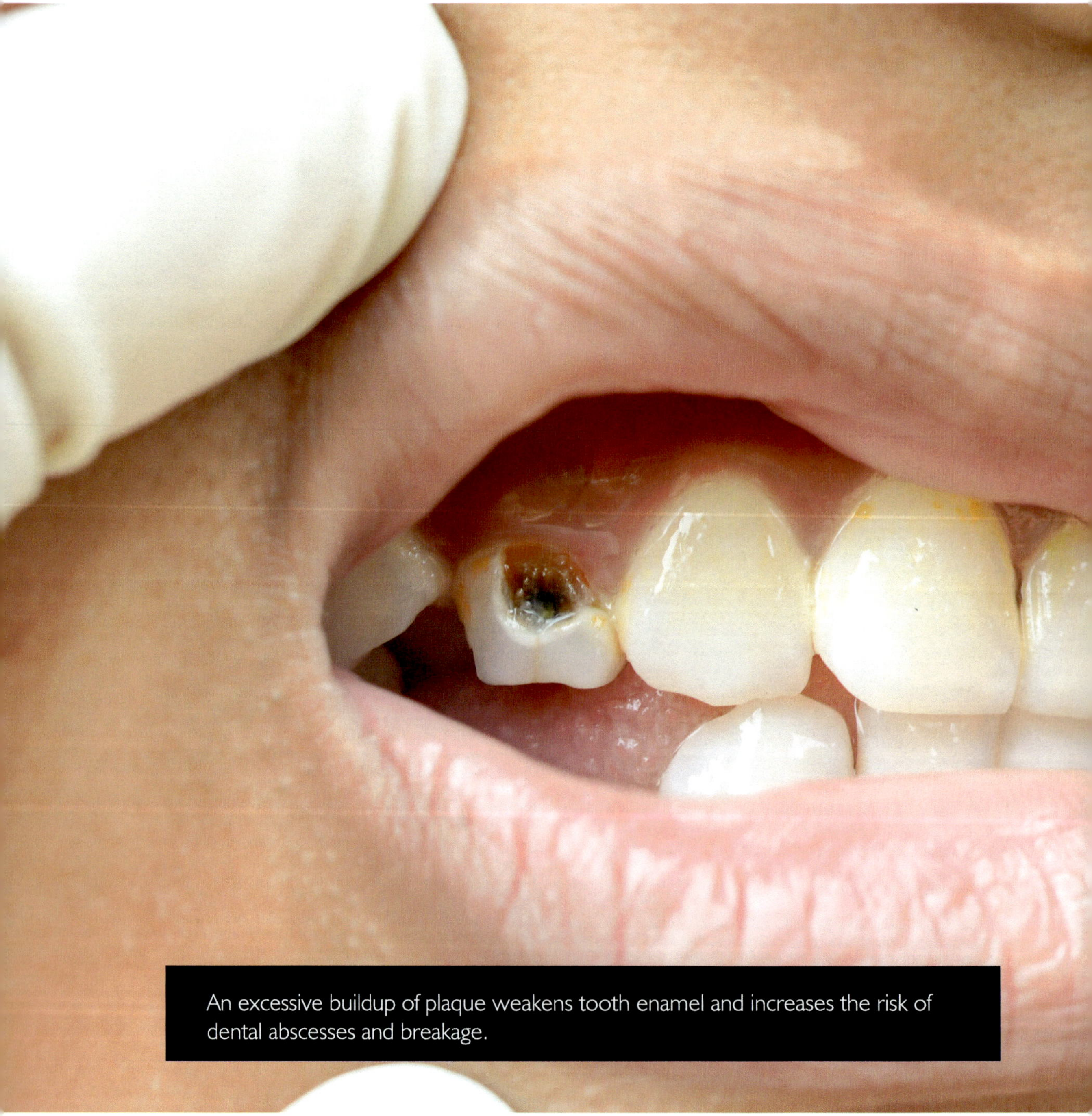

An excessive buildup of plaque weakens tooth enamel and increases the risk of dental abscesses and breakage.

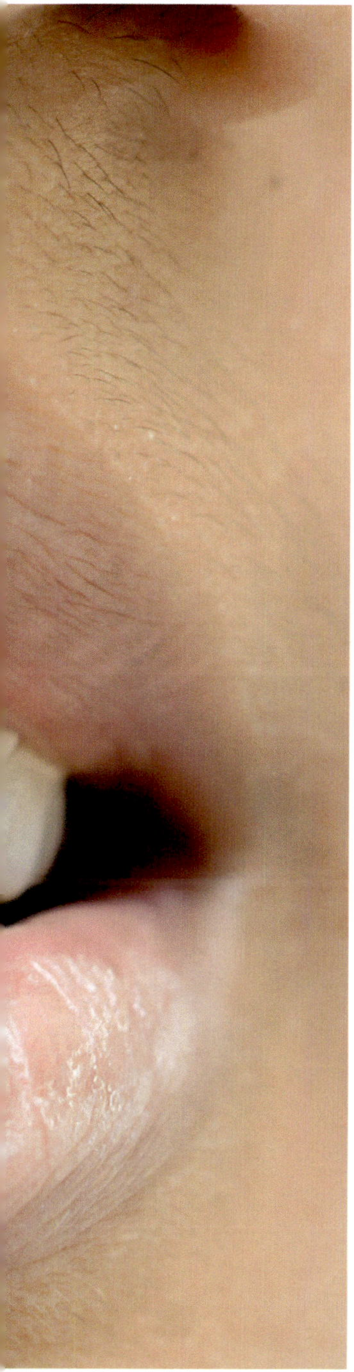

or flossing. A trip to the dentist will be necessary to remove it and stop the decay.

Despite increased efforts by organizations like the American Dental Association to spread awareness about good oral hygiene, cavities are still a growing problem. The results of a survey conducted by the National Institutes of Health (NIH) and the Centers for Disease Control and Prevention (CDC) revealed that 91 percent of US adults aged twenty to sixty-four had one or more cavities. Even more shocking was that more than a quarter of them hadn't sought any treatment for their cavities. Many children are affected by tooth decay as well, but the percentages are lower than for adults. Based on results from a previous survey, the NIH and CDC reported that 42 percent of US children aged two to eleven had cavities, with 23 percent of them not receiving treatment. Common cavity-causing culprits include poor oral hygiene, eating sticky, sugary foods, and a lack of fluoride in the water.

PREVENTING AND TREATING CAVITIES

Just like in the battle against bad breath, good oral hygiene plays the biggest role in successfully preventing tooth decay. Brushing and flossing and regular visits to the dentist are crucial to keep oral bacteria under control and prevent cavities. When a cavity does occur, it's important for a dentist to treat it as soon as possible, before the cavity grows larger. As long as the cavity hasn't rotted away too much of the tooth, a dentist can stop it from advancing by filling the cavity. There are several different

BEAUTIFUL BLACK TEETH

Although most people associate black teeth with tooth decay and cavities, in some parts of the world people dyed their teeth black because they thought it was beautiful. In Japan, this process was called ohaguro, and it was common for women to engage in this practice until the end of the nineteenth century. The process involved drinking a black liquid made from bits of iron soaked in vinegar. Unsurprisingly, it was said to taste terrible. In order to keep their teeth beautifully blackened, the women had to drink the liquid every day or at least every couple of days. Around the time ohaguro became popular, white faces, achieved by applying white makeup made from rice flour, were considered very desirable. Because of the white makeup, often women's teeth looked dramatically yellow. This problem was solved with ohaguro. In some parts of the world, such as remote, rural areas in Southeast Asia, the Pacific Islands, and South America, people still blacken their teeth. Ironically, even though black teeth are a sign of tooth decay, scientists have discovered that the coating used for blackening teeth actually provided some protection from rot and decay.

materials that can be used to fill a cavity, depending on which tooth the cavity is in, how deep the cavity is, and whether or not the patient has allergies to any of the filling materials. The dentist will first numb the area around the tooth and then remove the rotted area with a laser or drill. The cavity will then be filled with gold, amalgam, composite resin, or porcelain. If the tooth has fractured because of the cavity or if the decay has reached the nerve under the tooth, a more intense procedure, such as the removal of the nerve or a root canal, may be required. In extreme cases, the entire tooth may need to be extracted.

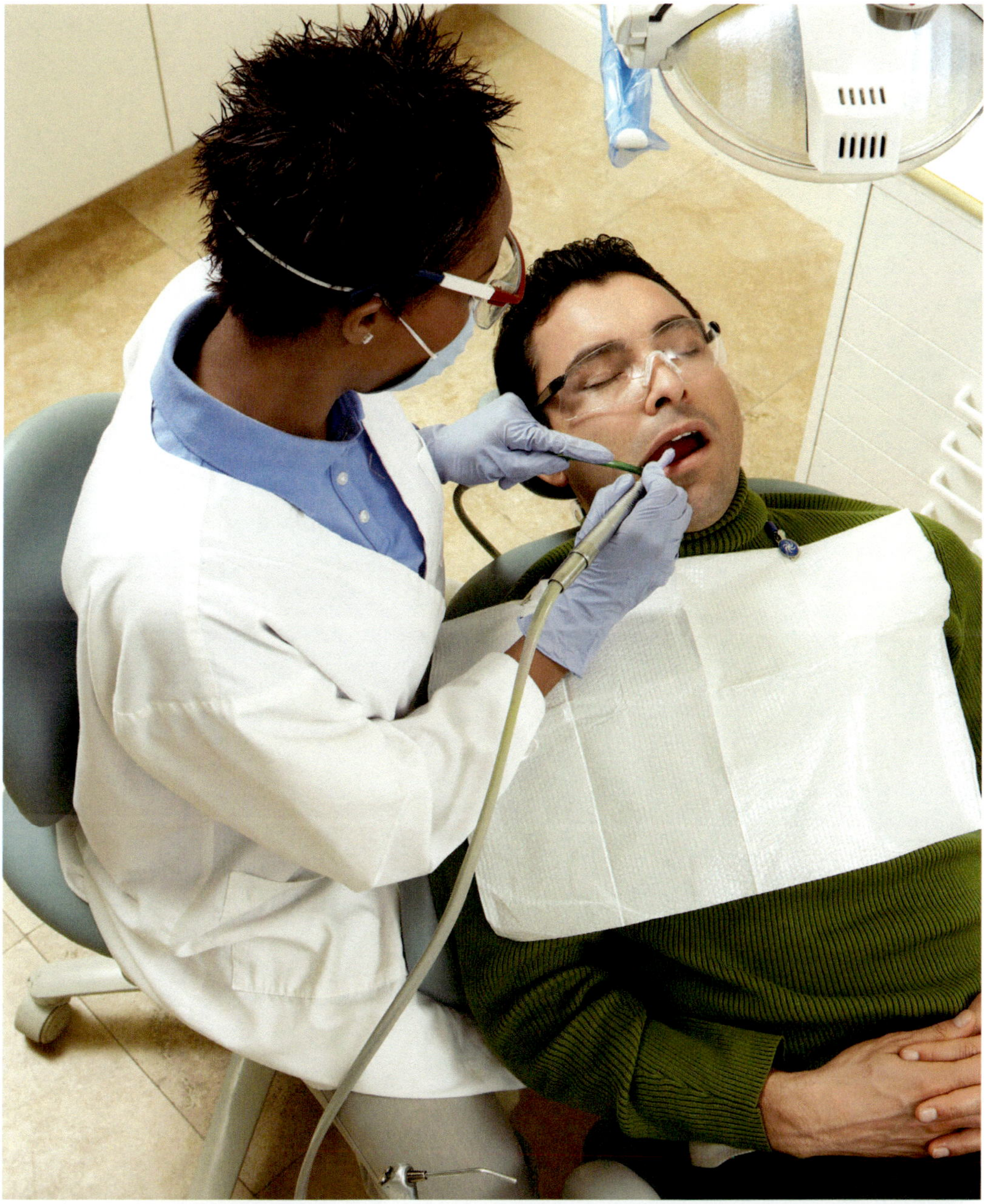

When a cavity is caught early enough, a dentist can stop it in its tracks, cleaning out the rotted area and using a special material to fill the cavity.

When plaque and tartar are left untreated, they not only cause cavities, they also cause gum disease. As gum disease progresses, pockets form between the gum and tooth. When the pockets become infected by bacteria, the condition is called periodontitis. Periodontitis can cause damage to the bones and tissues that hold teeth in place.

Cavities are associated with pain and discolored, rotting teeth, especially as they advance. When left untreated, though, the results can be far worse. Untreated cavities can lead to death. Two tragic cases in the United States involved a twelve-year-old boy and a twenty-six-year-old man. Both of them had untreated cavities that eventually caused a serious infection, which spread to their blood and brain. Despite antibiotic treatment when the pain became unbearable, the infection could not be stopped. Sadly, they both lost their lives because of a cavity.

MYTHS AND FACTS

Myth: Sugar is the main cause of cavities.
Fact: Sugar itself does not cause cavities. Cavities are formed when bacteria in the mouth produce acid that then attacks the teeth. The bacteria in the mouth that lead to cavities often come from foods rich in carbohydrates, such as potatoes, bread, rice, and even fruits and vegetables.

Myth: When someone has a cavity, he or she can feel it.
Fact: Though cavities are associated with tooth pain, until a cavity becomes advanced, reaching all the way down to the nerve of the tooth, there is often no pain. This is one reason why it is so important to get regular dental checkups—to catch those cavities before they become a real pain!

Myth: Children get cavities more frequently than adults.
Fact: There has actually been an increase in the number of adults and senior citizens with cavities and a decrease in the number of children with cavities. This is most likely due to the use of sealants (a thin, protective plastic coating) on children's teeth and increased awareness of the importance of regular visits to the dentist. Unfortunately, sometimes adults forget that it is just as important for them to have their teeth cleaned regularly as it is for children.

CHAPTER FOUR

GEOGRAPHY AND GENETICS: OTHER FACTORS IN ORAL HEALTH

For some people, it's not easy to make regular visits to a dentist. Where a person lives plays a big role in determining whether or not he or she has access to dental care. Another factor that makes someone more or less likely to have oral health problems lies in his or her chromosomes. Every person's unique genetic code is a blueprint of traits that that person has inherited, including the tendency to have few problems with one's teeth, or many, along with other health issues.

DENTAL HYGIENE AROUND THE WORLD

In industrialized countries like the United States, there is no shortage of dentists. Though it may take longer to get to a dentist for those who live in very rural areas, virtually any town or city large enough to have a grocery store will have a dental office. Finding a dentist in a developing country is a much harder—sometimes impossible—task. According to the FDI World Dental Federation, there is an average of one dentist for every 5,000 people in industrialized countries like the United States. In Africa, there is only one dentist for every 150,000 people. In other

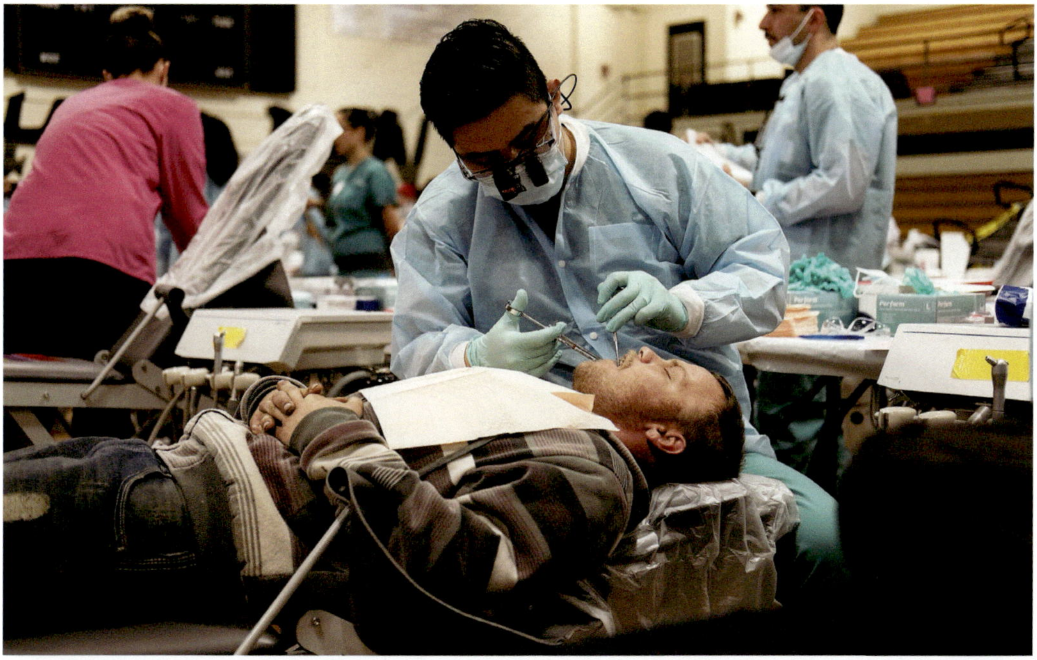

For many people in impoverished or remote areas around the world, free mobile clinics provide dental care that they would otherwise have to go without.

developing countries, such as India and Brazil, there are enough dentists, but they all tend to work in urban areas.

Visiting a dentist is a hardship for the many people in those countries who live far from a city and are struggling financially. A large percentage of the people in developing countries don't receive any dental care and are uneducated about even the most basic oral hygiene. Some don't even have clean water, toothpaste, or a toothbrush. The fact that it's so hard to get to a dentist in many of these countries means that by the time someone does manage to, the only option left for the dentist is usually to pull out their troubled tooth. In the African country of Tanzania, up to 90 percent of all dental work done is tooth extractions. Without regular dental checkups and treat-

NUTTY SCIENCE

In the quest for a clean, odor-free mouth, people around the world have tried many methods and products. Two of the most popular choices for fighting bad breath are mouthwash and chewing gum. Unfortunately, they cover up bad breath only temporarily and can be difficult to find in some parts of the world. In the African country of Nigeria, people spend a lot of money importing these types of products. Two teen scientists in Nigeria made a surprising discovery that may help many people have better oral hygiene. Eveshorhema Samuel-Alli, fourteen, and Ibukunoluwa Oladeinde, sixteen, students in Lagos, Nigeria, found that eating nuts from the African walnut tree prevented bad breath. After eating the walnuts one evening on a visit to a rural village, Eveshorhema was surprised to discover she had fresh breath in the morning, even before brushing her teeth. She remembered she had eaten walnuts the night before and ate more walnuts again that night. The results were the same the next morning. The two girls worked together to test the theory that the walnuts reduced bacteria and freshened breath. They divided volunteers into four groups. One group ate the walnuts, one chewed a special gum made from the walnuts, one rinsed with a mouthwash made from the walnuts, and one group—the control group—didn't use walnuts in any form. The results of their study showed that the control group had a lot of bacteria that caused bad breath in their mouths, and the three walnut groups had far less. The girls believe that certain chemicals in the walnuts, such as oleic acid, alkaloids, and tannins, killed off the bacterial microbes that cause bad breath. Their discovery means that people living in countries where the African walnut tree grows will no longer be dependent solely on imported products to deal with bad breath.

ment, oral infections are common and cavities eat away at teeth until they are completely rotted.

Even in industrialized countries with enough dentists to serve the entire population, the cost of dental care keeps many people from visiting a dentist. According to an annual US Survey of Dental Care Affordability and Accessibility, a large number of Americans see a dentist only when something is wrong, and more than 50 percent of Americans who don't have dental insurance don't get any preventive dental care whatsoever. When asked why they had delayed or skipped dental treatment, the number-one reason given was high costs. Preventive care can be expensive, especially without dental insurance, but it is far less expensive than the procedures that are required once there is a problem.

INHERITING TOOTH TROUBLE

Good dental hygiene is essential to having a healthy, cavity-free mouth, but genetics also play a role in tooth decay. In fact, a shocking 60 percent of the risk for tooth decay is determined by genetics. Scientists have discovered that genes play a role in tooth decay in five specific ways.

Whether a person craves sweets or is not that crazy about them is determined by their genetic "sweet preference." Those who have inherited a love of sweets are much more likely to develop tooth decay, even if they practice good oral hygiene.

Enamel is the protective, outer layer of teeth. Genetics determine how soft or hard the layer of enamel is. The softer the enamel is, the easier it is for bacteria to eat through a tooth's surface and cause a cavity.

The third area where genes play a role in tooth decay is referred to as "taste ability." Some people have greater sensitivity to flavors than others and can taste a greater variety of things. Studies have shown that the greater the variety in taste ability, the less likely a person is to develop tooth decay.

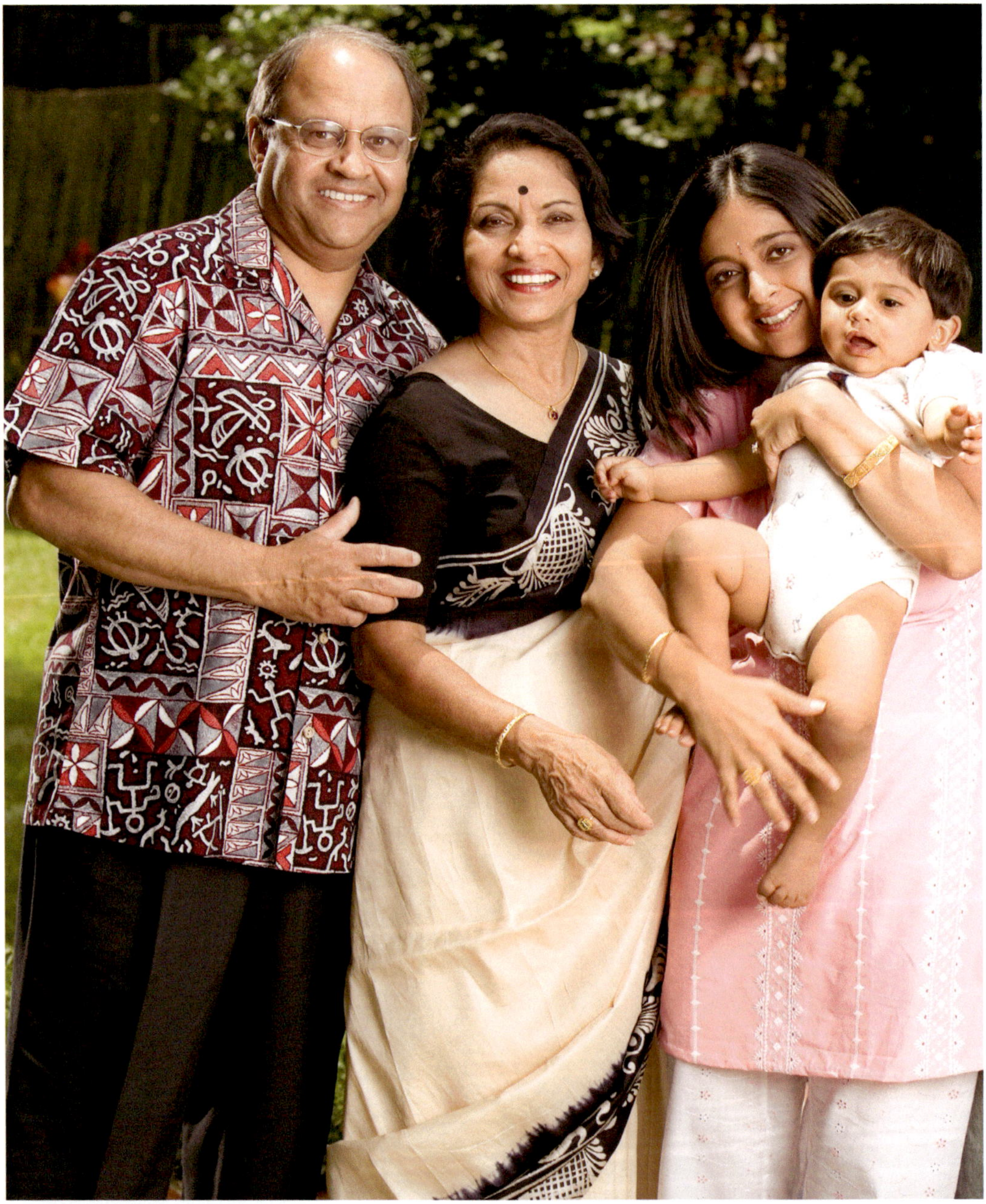

A healthy mouth that tends to be resistant to tooth decay—or a mouth that is especially vulnerable to tooth decay—is an inherited trait.

Vitamins and minerals in foods must be broken down when eaten in order to benefit the body. Saliva is an important part of that breakdown process, and the strength of saliva is determined by genetics. The better a person's saliva is at metabolizing the elements that strengthen teeth, the less likely a person is to have tooth decay.

There are many different communities of bacteria that live in the body. Several of them live in the mouth, on the tongue, the surface of the teeth, and below the gumline. Together, these communities of bacteria are called the microbiome. Everybody's immune system responds differently to his or her microbiome, based on genetics, and the way a person's immune system responds influences how likely that person is to have tooth decay.

Genes are responsible for approximately 60 percent of cavities, but diet, oral hygiene, tobacco use, access to dental care, culture, and finances account for the other 40 percent, according to Robert J. Weyant, chairman of the University of Pittsburgh's Department of Dental Public Health. Scientists believe frequent consumption of sugary drinks is the biggest environmental threat to dental health, while fluoride, whether in toothpaste, dental treatments, or the water supply, is the environmental factor most likely to help prevent tooth decay.

CHAPTER FIVE

BEYOND A CLEAN MOUTH: THE BENEFITS OF GOOD DENTAL CARE

Everyone appreciates a healthy, beautiful smile, and many people go to great lengths to care for their teeth in order to make sure they have one. A beautiful smile is a worthy goal, but there are many other important reasons to make good dental care a priority. Though some people dread a trip to the dentist, the risk of serious health problems that can arise from a lack of dental care should motivate them to do their best to take care of their teeth. Gone are the days when people had valid reasons to fear a trip to the dentist. Modern-day dentistry has made the experience of sitting in the dental chair easier and more pleasant than ever before.

GATEWAY TO THE BODY

Failing to regularly brush, floss, and get dental checkups allows nasty bacteria to take over the mouth, causing bad breath, cavities, gum disease, and oral infections. There is solid evidence, however, that people who neglect their teeth are putting themselves at risk for more than just oral health problems. Studies have found a strong link between a lack of good dental care and a variety of serious health outcomes. When harmful bac-

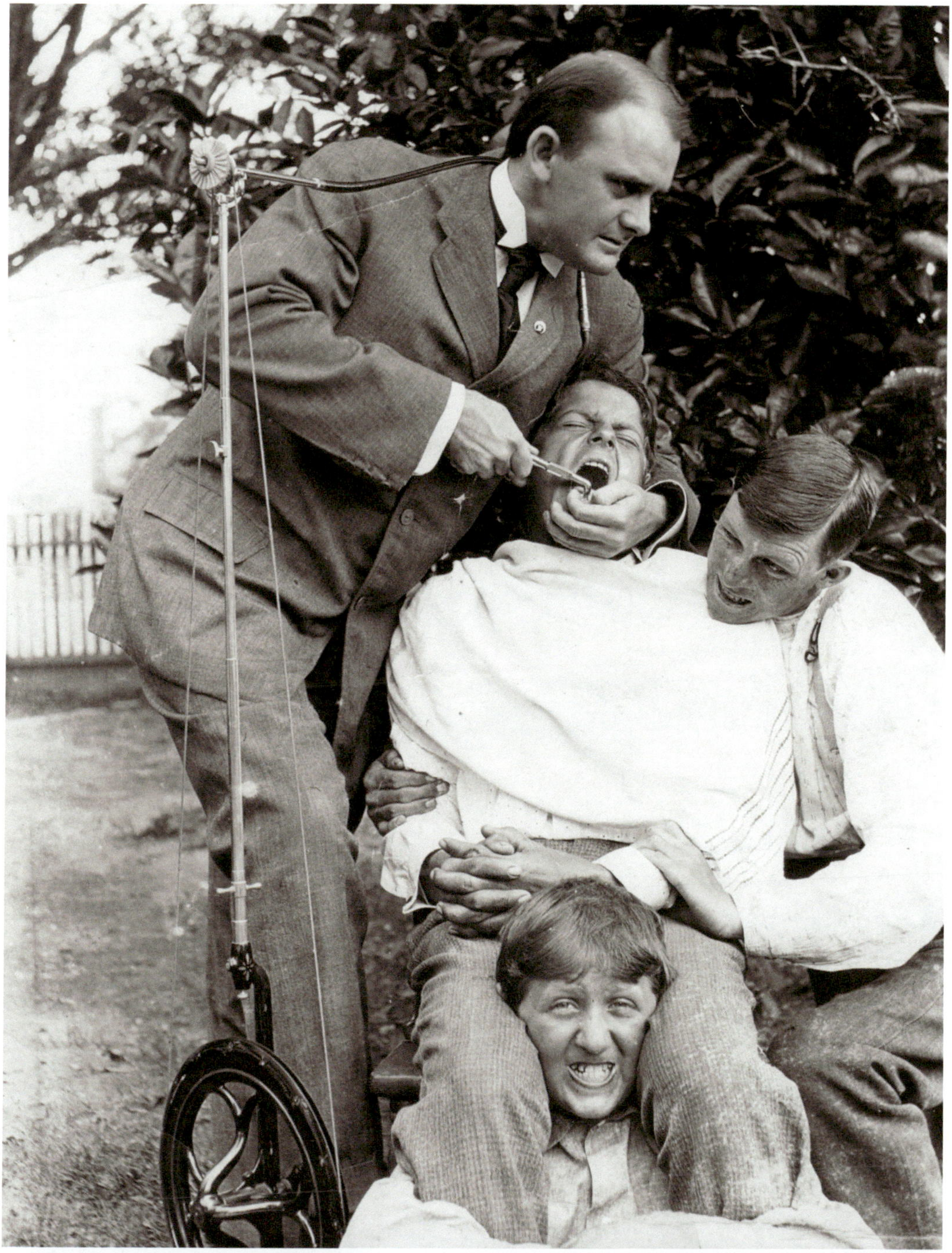

In the not-too-distant past, a trip to the dentist was often a very painful experience, and one that most people put off as long as possible.

teria build up on the teeth and gums, the bacteria eventually make their way into the bloodstream, where they can cause infections and illnesses throughout the body that have the potential to be deadly. Three of the most serious conditions linked to poor dental care are heart disease, diabetes, and respiratory infections.

Most people are aware that heart disease is a serious condition, but few are aware that gum disease or periodontitis can cause heart disease. When harmful bacteria in the mouth enter the bloodstream and make their way to arteries in the heart, they cause the arteries to form plaque on their inner walls. The plaque hardens the arteries and makes it difficult for blood to get through, which can cause heart attacks, strokes, and even death.

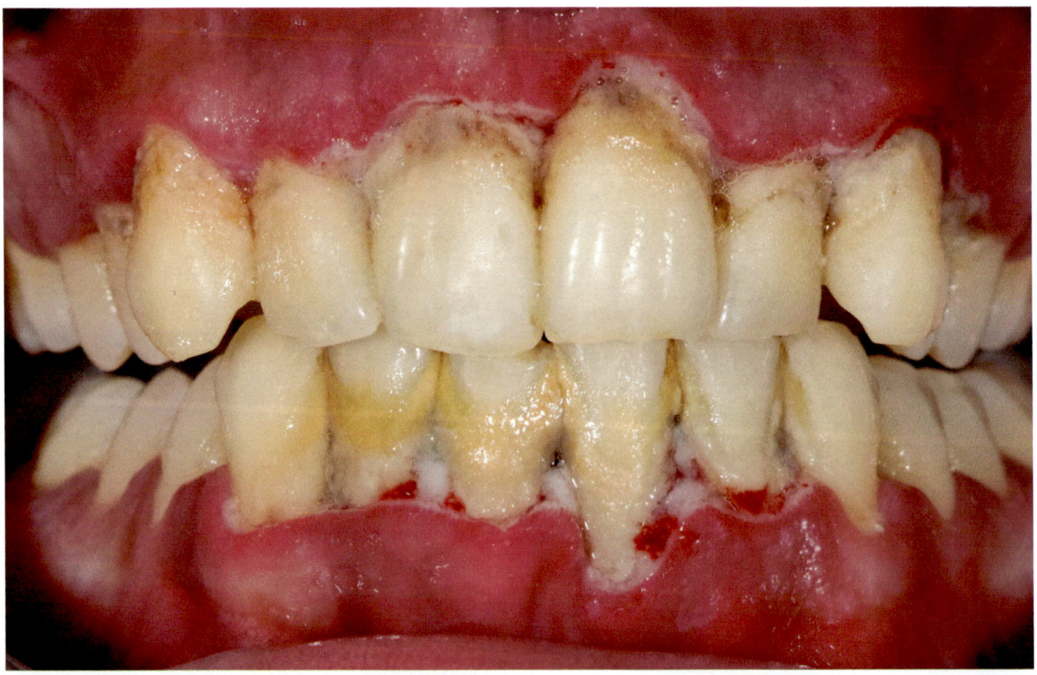

Left unchecked, plaque spreads to all surfaces of the teeth, hardens, and leads to tooth decay, gum disease, and many other illnesses.

Scientists have discovered that advanced gum disease causes higher blood sugar levels. High blood sugar puts people at risk of developing type 2 diabetes. For individuals who already have diabetes, gum disease makes it even more difficult for them to keep their blood sugar under control, which can lead to serious complications.

There are two ways oral bacteria can cause respiratory infections, like pneumonia. Infections can occur when bacteria enter the bloodstream and travel to the lungs or when a person repeatedly inhales bacteria from his or her infected teeth and gums. These infections can result in lengthy hospital stays and sometimes death.

In addition to these illnesses, scientists suspect that poor dental care may be linked to the onset of dementia or Alzheimer's disease. Harmful

DENTAL ASSISTANT OR DENTAL HYGIENIST?

Dental assistants and dental hygienists both play important roles at the dentist's office, but they have different training and job duties. It typically takes one to two years for dental assistants to complete training and become certified. Duties they perform may include taking X-rays, assisting the dentist with procedures, teaching patients about oral hygiene, preparing and sterilizing dental equipment, and general office management duties. Dental hygienists must have at least a two-year degree in dental hygiene. The duties of a dental hygienist include collecting information about the patient's medical history, removing plaque and thoroughly cleaning and polishing patients' teeth, applying fluoride and decay preventatives, and administering local anesthetics to numb a patient's mouth. Dental hygienists have completed more advanced training than dental assistants and spend a great deal of time with patients.

bacteria in the mouth are also believed to be a contributing factor in many types of cancer. The mouth is a gateway to all other parts of the body and keeping it clean and healthy is essential.

SOOTHING TRENDS IN DENTISTRY

Many people still struggle with a fear of going to the dentist, but dental care has come a long way. Gentler methods of dentistry and advances in dental equipment are keeping patients comfortable during procedures that used to be uncomfortable or even painful. Increasingly, "gentle dentistry" is the trend. Laser dentistry is one of the newer gentle den-

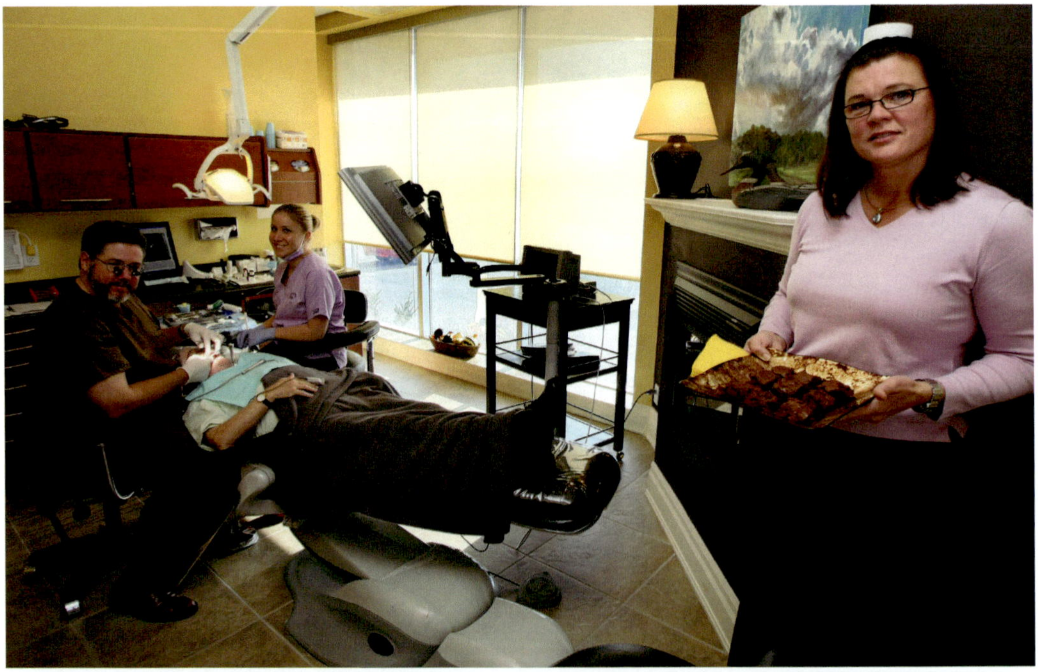

A soothing, comfortable environment and modern, gentle methods of dentistry have replaced the painful, frightening dental visits of the past.

tistry techniques. The technology behind the laser means that patients no longer have to experience the vibrations, heat, or pressure that used to be a part of dental procedures. The lasers are more accurate than the dental tools that were previously used, cause less bleeding and swelling, and reduce the risk of infection after a dental procedure. Another component of the new gentle dentistry trend is the use of things such as soothing music, movies, eye protection, massage chairs, and even pillows and blankets to keep patients calm and comfortable.

Hopefully, these advances in techniques and treatment methods will continue to encourage people to make and keep regular dental appointments.

Since the gross science behind the cause of bad breath and cavities has been uncovered, big improvements have been made in dental care. More and more people are becoming aware of the importance of good oral hygiene and regular dental visits, as well as the consequences of poor oral hygiene. As this knowledge spreads, the odds will increasingly be in favor of more healthy smiles that last a lifetime.

10 GREAT QUESTIONS TO ASK A DENTIST

1. When do adult teeth typically come in?
2. What kind of toothbrush should I use?
3. Should I use mouthwash every day?
4. What should I do if one of my teeth gets knocked out?
5. Why are my teeth sensitive to cold or hot?
6. What should I do if I have tooth pain?
7. Why do I need dental X-rays?
8. Am I brushing and flossing correctly?
9. Are my teeth and gums healthy?
10. When do I need to come back for my next visit?

GLOSSARY

amalgam A mixture of mercury and another metal, commonly used in dental fillings.

bacteria Tiny living organisms found everywhere that can be harmful or beneficial.

cavity The decayed part of a tooth.

control group The group in a study or experiment that does not receive treatment and is used to measure how the other groups in the study perform.

developing countries Countries that have little economic or industrial activity and where most people are living in poverty.

enamel The hard, outer layer of teeth.

extraction The action of removing something.

fluoride A natural mineral that helps to strengthen tooth enamel and is often added to drinking water.

halitosis The scientific term for bad breath.

industrialized countries Countries that have a highly developed economy and advanced industry and technology.

microbiome The group of microorganisms living in a particular environment together.

periodontitis An inflammation of the tissue around teeth that can cause the teeth to loosen.

plaque A sticky layer of bacteria on the teeth.

prophylactic Having to do with action taken to prevent disease.

root The soft part of a tooth below the surface that holds the tooth in place in the jaw.

saliva A clear liquid that keeps the mouth moist, helps fight germs in the mouth, protects tooth enamel, and aids in preventing tooth decay and gum disease.

tartar Hard deposits of plaque that form on the teeth.

FOR MORE INFORMATION

American Dental Association (ADA)
211 East Chicago Avenue
Chicago, IL 60611-2678
(312) 440-2500
Website: http://www.ada.org/en
Facebook: @AmericanDentalAssociation
Twitter: @AmerDentalAssn
Instagram: @americandentalassociation
The American Dental Association is the largest dental association in the United States and an excellent source of oral health related information for dentists and their patients.

American Dental Education Association (ADEA)
655 K Street NW
Suite 800
Washington, DC 20001
(202) 289-7201
Website: http://www.adea.org
Facebook: @ADEAweb
Twitter: @adeaweb
This organization promotes dental education and encourages individuals and institutions to address contemporary oral health-care issues.

American Dental Hygienists' Association (ADHA)
444 North Michigan Avenue
Suite 400
Chicago, IL 60611
(312) 440-8900
Website: http://www.adha.org
Facebook: @youradha
Twitter: @YourADHA
Instagram: @youradha

This organization provides information on advances in dental hygiene and offers the latest in training and information for dental hygienists. They are committed to improving the public's oral health.

Canadian Dental Association (CDA)
1815 Alta Vista Drive
Ottawa, Ontario, Canada
K1G 3Y6
(613) 523-1770
Website: https://www.cda-adc.ca/en/index.asp
Facebook: @CanadianDentalAssociation
Twitter: @CdnDentalAssoc
The Canadian Dental Association is a national organization in Canada devoted to promoting oral health and advancing the profession of dentistry.

Centers for Disease Control and Prevention (CDC)
1600 Clifton Road
Atlanta, GA 30329-4027
(800) 232-4636
Website: https://www.cdc.gov/oralhealth/index.html
Facebook: @cdc
Twitter: @cdcgov
Instagram: @cdcgov
The oral health division of the Centers for Disease Control and Prevention offers a wealth of information on topics such as proper oral care, water fluoridation, and state-sponsored oral health programs.

Office of Disease Prevention and Health Promotion
1101 Wootton Parkway, LL-100
Rockville, MD 20852
(240) 453-8281

Website: https://www.healthypeople.gov/2020/topics-objectives/topic/oral-health
Facebook: @HPDPmalta
Twitter: @gohealthypeople
The goal of this organization is to promote better health practices, including better oral health, for everyone. They offer information on preventive care, emerging issues in oral health, fluoridated water sources, and school-based dental sealant programs.

Ontario Dental Association
4 New Street
Toronto, ON M5R 1P6
(416) 922-3900
Website: http://www.youroralhealth.ca/index.php
Facebook: @OntarioDentalAssociation
Twitter: @ONDentalAssn
This organization is committed to the oral health of residents in Ontario, acts as the voice of Ontario dentists, and promotes advances in the field of dentistry.

FOR FURTHER READING

Allison, Linda, Rebecca Smith, and Judy Diamond. *Watch Your Mouth: Discover What's Alive Inside! The Amazing Microworld of Tongue Fuzz and Bad Breath.* Altadena, CA: Bitingduck Press, 2016.

Barnett, Richard. *The Smile Stealers: The Fine and Foul Art of Dentistry.* New York, NY: Thames & Hudson, 2017.

Guerini, Vincenzo. *A History of Dentistry from the Most Ancient Times Until the End of the Eighteenth Century.* London, UK: Forgotten Books, 2015.

Huey, Lois Miner. *Ick! Yuck! Eew! Our Gross American History.* Minneapolis, MN: Millbrook Press, 2014.

MacDonald, Fiona. *You Wouldn't Want to Live Without Dentists!* Danbury, CT: Franklin Watts, 2015.

Malaspina, Ann. *Tooth Traditions around the World.* North Mankato, MN: The Child's World, Inc., 2014.

Otto, Mary. *Teeth: The Story of Beauty, Inequality, and the Struggle for Oral Health in America.* New York, NY: The New Press, 2017.

Ungar, Peter S. *Evolution's Bite: A Story of Teeth, Diet, and Human Origins.* Princeton, NJ: Princeton University Press, 2017.

Ungar, Peter S. *Teeth: A Very Short Introduction.* Oxford, UK: Oxford University Press, 2014.

VanVoorst, Jenny Fretland. *Take a Closer Look at Your Teeth.* North Mankato, MN: The Child's World, Inc., 2014.

BIBLIOGRAPHY

Best Health Magazine Canada. "5 Foods That Fight Bad Breath." February 24, 2016.

http://www.besthealthmag.ca/best-you/oral-health/five-foods-treatments-for-bad-breath.

Brookshire, Bethany. "Solving Bad Breath One Walnut at a Time." Science News for Students, Society for Science and the Public. May 15, 2014.

http://www.sciencenewsforstudents.org/blog/eureka-lab/solving-bad-breath-one-walnut-time.

Brown, Peter. "Ohaguro." Ohaguro Tooth Staining in Edo Japan. Retrieved August 26, 2017.

http://www.peterbrown-palaeoanthropology.net/Ohaguro.html.

Drake, Nadia, et al. "The Evolution of Cavities." Phenomena, *National Geographic*. December 21, 2012.

http://phenomena.nationalgeographic.com/2012/12/21/the-evolution-of-cavities.

Fox, Maggie. "Who Has Cavities? Just about Everyone, Study Finds." TODAY.com. May 13, 2015.

http://www.today.com/health/most-us-have-tooth-decay-study-finds-t20781.

Franklin, Deborah. "To Beat Bad Breath, Keep the Bacteria in Your Mouth Happy." *Scientific American*, May 1, 2013.

http://www.scientificamerican.com/article/beat-bad-breath-keep-mouth-bacteria-happy.

Frysh, Paul. "Good or Bad Teeth? The Genetics of Tooth Decay." CNN, July 3, 2014.

http://www.cnn.com/2014/07/03/health/tooth-decay-causes/index.html.

Handwerk, Brian. "The History and Science Behind Your Terrible Breath." Smithsonian.com, February 13, 2017.

http://www.smithsonianmag.com/science-nature/halitosis-horrors-how-bad-breath-became-americas-worst-nightmare-180962104.

Jarus, Owen. "Mummy with Mouthful of Cavities Discovered." LiveScience, October 9, 2012.
http://www.livescience.com/23840-egyptian-mummy-cavities-death.html.

Lehman, Eric. "Alfred Fones, Irene Newman, and the Dental Hygiene Revolution." Bridgeport History Center. Retrieved August 15, 2017.
http://bportlibrary.org/hc/education/dr-alfred-fones.

Minutaglio, Rose, and Katherine Richter. "Complications from Tooth Infection Lead to California Father's Death." PEOPLE.com, February 3, 2017.
http://people.com/human-interest/complications-from-tooth-infection-leads-to-california-fathers-death.

Newman, Tim. "Bad Breath (Halitosis): Causes, Diagnosis and Treatment." Medical News Today, March 15, 2016.
http://www.medicalnewstoday.com/articles/166636.php.

Otto, Mary. "The Healthcare Gap: How Can a Child Die of Toothache in the US?" The Guardian, June 13, 2017.
http://www.theguardian.com/inequality/2017/jun/13/healthcare-gap-how-can-a-child-die-of-toothache-in-the-us.

Prichard, Denise. "A Brief History of the Toothbrush." Spear Education, March 15, 2013. http://www.speareducation.com/spear-review/2013/03/a-brief-history-of-the-toothbrush.

Sandilands, Tracey. "Top 10 Dental Questions You Should Ask." 10 Dental Questions You Should Ask | Colgate® Oral Care, January 12, 2016.
http://www.colgate.com/en/us/oc/oral-health/basics/dental-visits/article/top-10-dental-questions-you-should-ask-1015.

Watson, Traci. "Tooth Decay First Ravaged Human Society 15,000 Years Ago." *USA Today*, January 9, 2014.
http://www.usatoday.com/story/news/nation/2014/01/06/tooth-decay-archaeology/4307319.

Youn, Anthony. "What to Do about Your Bad Breath." CNN, February 22, 2014. http://www.cnn.com/2014/02/20/health/youn-bad-breath/index.html.

INDEX

ABOUT THE AUTHOR

Jessica Shaw holds a BA in psychology from Texas State University. She has worked in human services and as a preschool teacher. She writes nonfiction, fiction, and poetry for children and young adults, including standardized testing material and work appearing in numerous children's publications.

PHOTO CREDITS

Cover Zametalov/Shutterstock.com; cover, pp. 7, 13, 19, 26, 32 (background) Tatiana Shepeleva/Shutterstock.com; pp. 1, 4–5 (background) matthew25/Shutterstock.com; p. 5 Ira Block/NATIONAL GEOGRAPHIC IMAGE COLLECTION/Getty Images; p. 8 Leemage /Universal Images Group/Getty Images; p. 10 Heritage Images/Hulton Archive/Getty Images; p. 11 michaeljung/Shutterstock.com; p. 14 Jamesboy Nuchaikong/Shutterstock.com; p. 15 © iStockphoto.com /LeoPatrizi; p. 17 Medioimages/Photodisc/Thinkstock; pp. 20–21 © iStockphoto.com/Srisakorn; p. 23 Mike Watson Images/Moodboard /Thinkstock; p. 27 Spencer Platt/Getty Images; p. 30 Medioimages /Photodisc/Valueline/Thinkstock; p. 33 Transcendental Graphics/Archive Photos/Getty Images; p. 34 © iStockphoto.com/danielzgombic; p. 36 Ron Bull/Toronto Star/Getty Images.

Design: Michael Moy; Photo Researcher: Sherri Jackson